101 Testicular Cancer Juice and Meal Recipes:

The Solution to Testicular Cancer Using Vitamin Rich Foods

By

Joe Correa CSN

COPYRIGHT

This publication is designed to provide accurate and authoritative information in regard to the subject matter covered. It is sold with the understanding that neither the author nor the publisher is engaged in rendering medical advice. If medical advice or assistance is needed, consult with a doctor. This book is considered a guide and should not be used in any way detrimental to your health. Consult with a physician before starting this nutritional plan to make sure it's right for you.

ACKNOWLEDGEMENTS

This book is dedicated to my friends and family that have had mild or serious illnesses so that you may find a solution and make the necessary changes in your life.

101 Testicular Cancer Juice and Meal Recipes:

The Solution to Testicular Cancer Using Vitamin Rich Foods

By

Joe Correa CSN

CONTENTS

ABOUT THE AUTHOR

After years of Research, I honestly believe in the positive effects that proper nutrition can have over the body and mind. My knowledge and experience has helped me live healthier throughout the years and which I have shared with family and friends. The more you know about eating and drinking healthier, the sooner you will want to change your life and eating habits.

Nutrition is a key part in the process of being healthy and living longer so get started today. The first step is the most important and the most significant.

INTRODUCTION

101 Testicular Cancer Juice and Meal Recipes: The Solution to Testicular Cancer Using Vitamin Rich Foods

By Joe Correa CSN

Health risks that lead to testicular cancer have not yet been discovered, but there are some general prevention guidelines everyone should know about. A Healthy lifestyle and early prevention are crucial factors in treating almost every disease. When we talk about a healthy lifestyle, a proper, well balanced, and highly nutritional diet is the first thing that should be discussed.

You have to understand that your body is such a powerful machine with an amazing ability to heal itself, which is exactly why you should give it the right tools through proper nutrition. The recipes in this book are based on ingredients known for their anti-inflammatory and anti-bacterial properties. Besides that, all of the recipes are loaded with vitamins and minerals to help you boost your immune system.

Fruits and vegetables are known as the healthiest foods in the world. They are the perfect tool to prevent almost all diseases. Recent studies in Italy show that people who eat seven servings of tomato per week are 60% less likely to get cancer than those who only had two servings.

Some well-known antioxidants like garlic, onions, and basil, are proven to prevent different types of cancer, including testicular cancer. Their amazing antimicrobial properties are the main reason I have chosen to include them in so many recipes in this book.

Another cancer-preventive superfood are berries! They are extremely high in bioflavonoids known as the strongest antioxidants. Recipes like "Blueberry Green Tea Smoothie" will boost your immune system and can clean your body of toxins in no time! It's a perfect option for a quick breakfast or an afternoon snack and will take just a few minutes to make!

This book includes meal and juice recipes that contain all the superfoods necessary to prevent testicular cancer and improve your overall health.

101 TESTICULAR CANCER JUICE AND MEAL RECIPES: THE SOLUTION TO TESTICULAR CANCER USING VITAMIN RICH FOODS

MEALS

1. Strawberry Muffins

Ingredients:

6 oz. of strawberries, halved

2 cups of all-purpose flour

3 tsp of baking powder

1 tbsp. of brown sugar

2 large eggs

1 cup of skim milk

1 medium-sized banana, sliced

6 tbsp. of cream cheese

¼ tsp of salt

Preparation:

Preheat the oven to 400°F.

Combine flour, baking powder, and sugar. In a separate bowl, whisk the eggs, milk, and banana. Stir in into dry ingredients.

Add strawberries and stir well again.

Grease the muffin mold and spoon in the mixture evenly. Top each muffin with a tablespoon of cream cheese and place it in the oven.

Bake for 25 minutes and remove from the heat. Leave it to cool for a while.

Nutritional information per serving: Kcal: 112, Protein: 4.2g, Carbs: 19.7g, Fats: 1.4g

2.   Zucchini Oven Fried Rings

Ingredients:

2 medium-sized zucchini, ringed

1 tbsp. of dried oregano, ground

1 tbsp. of cumin, ground

2 tbsp. of olive oil

Preparation:

Preheat the oven to 400°F.

Cut the zucchini into rings and spread over a baking sheet. Sprinkle with oregano and cumin to taste. Drizzle with olive oil and place into the oven.

Bake for 15 minutes.

Serve with tomato salsa or any other dipping you wish.

Nutritional information per serving: Kcal: 20, Protein: 1.2g, Carbs: 3.6g, Fats:2.2g

3.　　Blueberry Banana Smoothie

Ingredients:

1 cup of skim milk

¼ cup of frozen blueberries

1 large banana, sliced

2 tbsp. of flax seeds

Preparation:

Combine all ingredients in a blender. Blend for 2 minutes, or until smooth. Transfer to a serving glasses and refrigerate for 30 minutes before serving.

Nutritional information per serving: Kcal: 290, Protein: 11.3g, Carbs: 48.5g, Fats: 8.2g

4.   Salmon with Basil

Ingredients:

1 lb. of salmon fillets, skinless and boneless

12 oz. of broccoli

12 oz. baby carrots, whole

1 lemon, peeled and wedged

8 garlic cloves, crushed

1 tsp of salt

2 tbsp. of fresh basil, finely chopped

5 tbsp. of olive oil

Preparation:

Combine garlic, basil, salt, and pepper in a blender. Gradually add the oil and blend for 10 seconds each time (if you add too much oil at a time, it won't combine). Transfer the mixture in a dip bowl. Set aside.

Place carrots in a deep pot of boiling water. Cook for 5 minutes and then add broccoli. Cook for 3 minutes more and remove from the heat. Transfer to a serving plate. Season with some salt and pepper to taste.

Preheat 1 tablespoon of oil in a large frying skillet over a medium-high temperature. Place in the meat and season with some salt and pepper. Cook for 3 to 4 minutes from both sides, or until doneness. Remove from the heat and transfer to a serving plate.

Drizzle the meat with garlic sauce and serve with vegetables and lemon wedges.

Nutrition information per serving: Kcal: 620, Protein: 46.3g, Carbs: 4.5g, Fats: 47.5g

5.   Orange and Chive Salad

Ingredients:

8 oranges, peeled and chopped

2 tbsp. of chives, finely chopped

1 cup of Romaine lettuce, chopped

1 garlic clove, minced

2 tbsp. of lemon juice

2 tbsp. of olive oil

1 tbsp. of fresh parsley, finely chopped

1 tbsp. of Dijon mustard

Preparation:

Combine garlic, mustard, oil, and lemon juice in a small mixing bowl. Whisk all well to combine. Set aside.

Place the oranges in a large salad bowl. Add the parsley and chives, and stir well. Pour the previously prepared dressing over the oranges and give it a finally stir. Line lettuce leaves on a serving plate and spoon the mixture equally.

Serve immediately.

Nutrition information per serving: Kcal: 397, Protein: 7.6g, Carbs: 88.4g, Fats: 1.8g

6.   Stuffed Tomatoes

Ingredients:

4 large tomatoes, whole

1 cup of Mozzarella cheese, crumbled

½ cup of onion, finely chopped

10 of spinach, finely chopped

2 tbsp. of Parmesan cheese, grated

1tbsp of fresh parsley, finely chopped

2 tbsp. of olive oil

½ tsp of salt

¼ tsp of black pepper, ground

Preparation:

Preheat the oven to 400°F.

Carefully place spinach in a pot of boiling water. Cook for 1 minute and remove from the heat. Drain well and set aside.

Hollow out the tomatoes and reserve the pulp. Remove the seeds out of pulp and chop it into a large mixing bowl. Stir in the spinach, Mozzarella, Parmesan, salt, and pepper.

Spoon the mixture into the tomatoes and place them into a previously greased baking dish. Bake for 5 minutes and remove from the heat.

Enjoy!

Nutrition information per serving: Kcal: 159, Protein: 14.5g, Carbs: 12.9g, Fats: 10.8g

7.   Pumpkin Oatmeal

Ingredients:

2 cups of oats, quick-cooking

3 cups of skim milk

½ cup of pumpkin, canned

½ tsp of cinnamon

¼ cup of raisins

1 tbsp. of chia seeds

Preparation:

Place the oats into a mixing bowl. Stir in the milk and put it into a microwave for 3 minutes.

Remove from the microwave and add all pumpkin and chia seeds. Stir well to combine and heat up for extra 40 seconds.

Top with raisings and serve.

Nutrition information per serving: Kcal: 272, Protein: 14.4g, Carbs: 47.5g, Fats: 3.6g

8.   Balsamic Berry Cucumber Salad

Ingredients:

1 cup of cucumber, sliced

1 cup of fresh blueberries

1 cup of red onion, sliced

½ cup of toasted almonds, chopped

1 cup of white quinoa

3 tbsp. of balsamic vinegar

1 tbsp. of honey

1 tbsp. of olive oil

Preparation:

Place quinoa in a medium-sized pot of boiling water. Reduce the heat and cover with a lid. Cook for about 10 to 15 minutes. Drain and transfer quinoa into a salad bowl to cool. Set aside.

Combine vinegar, honey and olive oil in a small mixing bowl. Whisk to combine and mix with quinoa.

Add blueberries, cucumber and red onion to the bowl. Sprinkle with toasted almonds and serve.

Nutrition information per serving: Kcal: 171, Protein: 5.5g, Carbs: 30.4g, Fats: 5.3g

9.   Lamb Chops in Garlic Sauce

Ingredients:

1 lb. of loin lamb chops

2 lbs. of green beans

2 tbsp. of garlic, minced

2 tbsp. of parsley, freshly minced

5 tbsp. of olive oil

1 tsp of red pepper, crushed

2 tbsp. of rosemary freshly minced

½ tsp of salt

Preparation:

Put the beans in a medium-sized pot of boiling water. Add a teaspoon of salt and cover with a lid. Reduce the temperature to low and cook for 15 minutes, or until fork-tender. Drain the beans and transfer to a serving bowl. Season with some salt and pepper, and drizzle with 2 tablespoons of olive oil. Stir well to combine. Set aside.

Combine garlic, parsley, rosemary, red pepper, and 2 tablespoons of olive oil in a small mixing bowl. Spread the mixture over the lamb chops.

Heat 1 tablespoon of olive oil in a frying skillet over a medium-high temperature. Place the lamb chops and cook for 4-5 minutes on each side or until nicely brown. Transfer the meat to a serving plate.

Serve with green beans, and if you like, you can add more vegetables.

Nutrition information per serving: Kcal: 192, Protein: 27.4g, Carbs: 55.3g, Fats: 13.7g

10.   Tomato & Chickpea Soup

Ingredients:

8 oz. of tomatoes, canned

1o oz. of chickpeas, pre-cooked

5 cups of chicken broth

1 medium-sized onion, sliced

1 tbsp. of fresh parsley, finely chopped

½ cup of white rice, uncooked

2 garlic cloves, minced

1 tsp of vegetable oil

½ tsp of salt

¼ tsp of black pepper, ground

Preparation:

Heat up the oil in a large frying pan over a medium-high temperature. Add the onions and stir-fry until translucent. Stir in tomatoes, garlic, and rosemary. Cook until remaining juices evaporate.

Now, add rice and broth. Bring it to a boil and then reduce the heat to low. Cover with a lid and simmer for about 10 to 15 minutes.

Add chickpeas and give it a final stir. Continue to cook for another 5 minutes. remove from the heat and stir in the parsley.

Serve warm.

Nutrition information per serving: Kcal: 371, Protein: 15.3g, Carbs: 64.2g, Fats: 5.8g

11.   Chicken with Lemon and Rosemary

Ingredients:

1 whole chicken, (3 lbs.)

1 cup of lemon juice

1 tsp if dried rosemary, ground

2 tbsp. of olive oil

½ tsp of salt

¼ tsp of black pepper, ground

¼ tsp of Cayenne pepper

¼ tsp of vegetable seasoning mix

Preparation:

Cut the chicken into two equal halves. Cut along the breast bone and back bone. Place the meat into a large marinade bowl. Add remaining ingredients and leave it to marinate for 2 hours to allow flavors to mingle. Using a tablespoon, coat the chicken with marinade frequently.

Meanwhile, preheat the grill to a medium heat. Transfer the meat to the grill and reserve the marinade. Cook for 10 minute on both sides then reduce to low. Using a kitchen brush, add marinade to the meat and cook for 10 minutes more or until done.

Serve the meat with steamed vegetables or sour cream.

Nutrition information per serving: Kcal: 55, Protein: 6.7g, Carbs: 3.2g, Fats: 4.7g

12.   Tomato and Peppers Omelet

Ingredients:

6 free-range eggs

1 large tomato, chopped

1 large bell pepper, chopped

1 tbsp. of olive oil

1 small onion, diced

2 oz. of mushrooms, halved

½ tsp of salt

¼ tsp of black pepper, ground

2 tbsp. of sour cream

¼ cup of cheddar cheese, crumbled

Preparation:

Preheat the oil in a large frying skillet over a medium-high temperature. add onion, mushrooms, and pepper. You can add 1-2 tablespoon of water to get more juicy mixture. Sauté for 5-6 minutes and add tomato. Cook for 5 minutes more and then add tomato. Set aside.

Combine eggs and sour cream in a mixing bowl. Whisk well to combine and set aside.

Now, preheat the remaining oil in a non-stick pan over a medium-high temperature. Pour in the eggs mixture and cook for 2 minutes. Now add the vegetables and cheese onto one half of the omelet. Fold the other half over and cook for 1-2 minutes, or until eggs are completely set.

Nutrition information per serving: Kcal: 264, Protein: 25.7g, Carbs: 8.6g, Fats: 13.8g

13. Swiss Steak

Ingredients:

1 lb. of round beef steak

3 tbsp. of all-purpose flour

2 tbsp. of olive oil

¼ cup of fresh celery, finely chopped

1 large carrot, diced

2 cups of tomato sauce

1 tbsp. of Worcestershire sauce

Preparation:

Preheat the oven to 400°F.

Place the meat into a large bowl and coat with flour.

Heat the oil in a large skillet over a medium-high temperature. cook the meat for 5 minutes on both sides, or until nicely brown. Transfer meat to a baking sheet and reserve the pan. Add all other ingredients to the pan and stir well to combine. Cook for 3 minutes and remove from the heat.

Pour the vegetables mixture over meat and cover with a lid. Reduce the temperature to low and bake until meat fork-tender.

Nutrition information per serving: Kcal: 308, Protein: 42.2g, Carbs: 9.5g, Fats: 10.3g

14.   Peach Smoothie

Ingredients:

½ cup of frozen peaches, sliced

½ cup of vanilla yogurt

1 cup of banana, sliced

¼ cup of orange juice

Preparation:

Combine all ingredients in a blender and blend until you get thick and creamy mixture. Transfer to the serving glasses and refrigerate at least 15 minutes before serving.

Nutrition information per serving: Kcal: 541, Protein: 18.1g, Carbs: 120.2g, Fats: 6.4g

15.   Cabbage Sprout Salad

Ingredients:

1 cup of red cabbage, shredded

2 medium-sized carrots, grated

2 cups of quinoa, pre-cooked

¼ cup of roasted almonds

½ cup of spring onions

1 small apple, grated

3 tbsp. of olive oil

1tbsp of apple cider vinegar

1tsp of honey

½ tsp of salt

Preparation:

Combine oil, vinegar, honey and salt in a mixing bowl. Stir well to combine and set aside for 10 minutes to allow flavors to mingle.

In a large serving bowl, combine cooked quinoa, cabbage, almonds, carrot, apple and onions. Drizzle with marinade and serve.

Nutrition information per serving: Kcal: 221, Protein: 5.2g, Carbs: 23.4g, Fats: 13.5g

16.　Chicken Breasts with Wild Mushrooms & Chestnuts

Ingredients:

1 lb. of chicken breasts, skinless and boneless

2 shallots, finely chopped

3 garlic cloves, crushed

1 cup of chicken broth

1 tsp of rosemary, finely chopped

1 tsp of cornstarch

1 tbsp. of balsamic vinegar

1 tbsp. of olive oil

For mushrooms:

1 lb. of wild mushrooms, halved

1 lb. of chestnuts, pre-cooked

1 tbsp. of fresh parsley, finely chopped

1 tbsp. of olive oil

½ tsp of salt

Preparation:

Heat up the oil in a non-stick frying pan over a medium-high temperature. Add mushrooms and cook for 5 minutes, and then add the chestnuts. Stir constantly and cook for 3 minutes more. Remove from the heat and cover to stay warm.

Heat the oil in a large frying skillet over a medium-high temperature. Add chicken and season with some salt and pepper to taste. Cook for 3 minutes on each side. Now, reduce the heat to low and add garlic, vinegar, and shallots. Add ½ cup of chicken broth, sprinkle with rosemary and bring it to a boil.

Reduce the heat and cover with a lid. Cook for 10 minutes or until chicken fork-tender. Remove the meat and transfer to the serving plate. Cover with aluminum foil to stay warm.

Add remaining broth to the pan and cook until liquid evaporates to 1 cup approximately. Stir in the cornstarch to get thicker mixture. Add parsley and bring it to a boil. Remove from the heat and pour over the meat on a serving plate.

Serve the juicy meat with previously prepared mushrooms and chestnuts.

utrition information per serving: Kcal: 238, Protein: 21.3g, Carbs: 17.9g, Fats: 10.4g

17.   Avocado Sandwich

Ingredients:

½ lb. turkey fillets, cut into strips

2 avocado slice, thinly sliced

½ cup of button mushrooms, halved

4 lettuce leaves, whole

3 tbsp. of olive oil

Preparation:

Cut turkey breast fillet into half inch strips. Heat up the olive oil in a large saucepan over a medium-high temperature. Reduce the temperature to low and cook for about 15 minutes.

Remove the turkey fillets from the saucepan and use a kitchen paper to remove the excess oil. Transfer to a plate.

Pour the olive oil from the saucepan and put the pan back to the heat. Slice the button mushrooms in half and add to the saucepan. Cook for about 3-4 minutes, over a medium heat, until all the water evaporates. Remove from the saucepan and allow it to cool for a while.

Use avocado slices to prepare a tasty sandwich.

Nutrition information per serving: Kcal: 378, Protein: 8.7g, Carbs: 43.2g, Fats: 20.6g

18.   Basil Eggs

Ingredients:

2 large eggs

1 tbsp. of fresh basil, finely chopped

¼ tsp of black pepper, ground

Preparation:

Add the eggs to a pot of boiling water. Be very gentle while doing this to prevent the eggs to crack.

One useful tip to prepare the perfect eggs is to add 1 tbsp. of baking soda into the boiling water. This will make a peeling process much easier.

Boil the eggs for 8 minutes. You can use a kitchen timer, or simply your watch. After 8 minutes, drain the water and place the eggs under the cold water for few minutes. Peel and slice the eggs. Sprinkle with chopped basil and serve.

Nutrition information per serving: Kcal: 160, Protein: 13.6g, Carbs: 3.8g, Fats: 9.5g

19. Beef Sirloin with Eggplant Slices

Ingredients:

1 beef sirloin, thinly sliced

1 medium-sized eggplant, peeled and cubed

1 tsp of olive oil

1 tbsp. of fresh basil, chopped

¼ tsp of pepper

Preparation:

Wash and pepper the meat.

Preheat the grill on a high temperature. Grill the meat on a barbecue pan for about 10 minutes on each side. Remove the meat and reserve the pan.

Peel the eggplant and cut into thick slices. Fry for few minutes in the reserved barbecue pan. Remove from heat and serve with beef.

Sprinkle with chopped basil.

Nutrition information per serving: Kcal: 416, Protein: 32.4g, Carbs: 30.1g, Fats: 15.3g

20.   Pineapple Omelet with Almonds

Ingredients:

3 thick slices of pineapple, peeled

2 free-range eggs

½ cup of almonds, minced

1 tbsp. of vegetable oil

½ tsp of salt

Preparation:

Break the eggs into a bowl and beat well until combined. Add minced almonds and mix well. Season with salt.

Heat up the oil in a large saucepan, over a medium temperature. Fist you want to fry pineapple slices for about 2-3 minutes on each side, until nicely golden brown color. Reduce the heat to low. Pour egg mixture into pan and fry for few more minutes, stirring constantly. Remove from the heat and enjoy.

Nutrition information per serving: Kcal: 174, Protein: 14.2g, Carbs: 8.5g, Fats: 10.6g

21.   Fruit salad

Ingredients:

1 cup of berries

½ cup of pineapple, cubed

½ cup of apple, chopped

5 mint springs

1 tbsp. of fresh lime juice

1 tsp of lime zest

¼ cup of water

1 tsp of cinnamon, ground

Preparation:

In a small saucepan combine ¼ cup of water, mint spring, fresh lime juice and lime zest. Allow it to boil over medium temperature and cook for about 2-3 minutes. Remove from the heat and cool.

Meanwhile, in a large bowl, combine 1 cup of berries, ½ cup of pineapple cubes and ½ cup of chopped apple. Pour the lime mixture over the salad and let it stand in the refrigerator for 20-30 minutes. Remove from the refrigerator and sprinkle with 1 tsp of cinnamon before serving.

Nutrition information per serving: Kcal: 164, Protein: 0.2g, Carbs: 42.5g, Fats: 0.4g

22.   Vanilla Rolls

Ingredients:

1 cup of almond flour

2 tbsp. of coconut flour

1 tsp of baking soda

2 tsp of vanilla extract

2 tbsp. of coconut oil

2 large eggs

1/3 cup of prunes, finely chopped

1/3 cup of almonds, minced

1 tsp of cinnamon

Preparation:

Preheat the oven to 325°F.

Mix together almond flour, coconut flour, baking soda and vanilla extract. Add the eggs and coconut oil. Whisk together until smooth mixture. Set aside.

In another bowl, combine the prunes, minced almonds, and cinnamon. Stir well.

Transfer the dough onto a baking sheet. Roll into a long rectangle and sprinkle with the plum mixture. Cut into 7 equal pieces and let it stand in the refrigerator for about 20 minutes before baking.

Bake the rolls for about 10 minutes, or until nice golden color.

Serve warm.

Nutrition information per serving: Kcal: 211, Protein: 12.7g, Carbs: 39.6g, Fats: 14.3g

23. Grilled Eggplant Slices with Chopped Fennel

Ingredients:

1 large eggplant

½ cup of fresh fennel, chopped

1 tbsp. of olive oil

1 tsp of fresh parsley, finely chopped

Preparation:

Peel the eggplant and cut into 3 equal slices. Bake it in a barbecue pan without oil. When done, spread olive oil over it, sprinkle with fennel and parsley.

(These eggplant slices are great cold, so you can leave them overnight in a refrigerator)

Nutrition information per serving: Kcal: 101, Protein: 1.2g, Carbs: 8.2g, Fats: 9.3g

24.   Watermelon Smoothie

Ingredients:

2 cups of watermelon, cubed

¼ cup of milk, fat-free

1 tbsp. of chia seeds

1 tsp of fresh mint, ground

Preparation:

Combine all ingredients in a blender. Blend for 20 seconds, and add few ice cubes. Blend for 30 seconds more and transfer to the serving glasses.

Top with mint and serve.

Nutrition information per serving: Kcal: 186, Protein: 5.8g, Carbs: 24.2g, Fats: 9.3g

25. Cinnamon Cookies

Ingredients:

1 cup of almonds, whole

½ cup of cashews

½ cup of all-purpose flour

2 tbsp. of honey

1 large egg

1 egg white

2 tbsp. of butter

2 tbsp. of cornstarch

1 tsp of cinnamon

Preparation:

Preheat the oven to 325°F.

Combine almonds and cashews in a food processor. Blend for 2 minutes and add flour, butter, cinnamon, cornstarch, egg, egg white, and honey. Pulse for another 2 minutes. Transfer the dough to a clean working space and form the cookies.

Line a baking sheet with a parchment and place the cookies. Make about 1 inch space between them.

Bake for 15 minutes, or until nicely golden brown. Remove from the oven and place on a rack to cool for a while.

Serve with a green or black tea.

Nutrition information per serving: Kcal: 33, Protein: 0.2g, Carbs: 4.2g, Fats: 0.8g

26.   Turkey Fillet with Walnuts

Ingredients:

3 turkey fillets

½ cup of walnuts

¼ cup of water

1 tbsp. of olive oil

½ tsp of salt

Preparation:

Fry the fillets in a barbecue pan, over a low temperature, for about 15 minutes, or until tender. Remove the pan from the heat and add water and walnuts. Mix well and fry for another 5-6 minutes until the water evaporates. Stir constantly. Allow it to cool for a while before serving.

Nutrition information per serving: Kcal: 82, Protein: 13.5g, Carbs: 4.5g, Fats: 6.7g

27.   Nutmeg Omelet

Ingredients:

3 large eggs

1 medium-sized onion, diced

2 tbsp. of olive oil

1 tsp of nutmeg

¼ tsp of salt

¼ tsp of black pepper, ground

Preparation:

Peel and slice the onion. Wash under the cool water and drain. Set aside.

Heat the olive oil in a nonstick skillet over a medium-high temperature.

In a small bowl, whisk together eggs and pepper. Pour the eggs in a skillet and fry for about 3 minutes. Using a spatula, remove the eggs from the frying pan and add onions and nutmeg. Stir well and return the eggs to the skillet.

Cook for few more minutes, until the onions get nice golden color. Remove from the heat and serve!

Nutrition information per serving: Kcal: 223, Protein: 19.2g, Carbs: 10.2g, Fats: 38.4g

28.   Smooth Banana with Honey

Ingredients:

1 large banana

2 egg whites

1.5 cup of coconut milk

1 tbsp. of raw honey

1 tsp of ground vanilla

Preparation:

Peel and chop the banana into small cubes. Combine with other ingredients in a blender and mix for 30 seconds, until smooth mixture. Keep in the refrigerator and serve cold.

Nutrition information per serving: Kcal: 248, Protein: 13.6g, Carbs: 27.9g, Fats: 10.1g

29.   Almond Waffles

Ingredients:

½ cup of almond flour

¼ cup of coconut flour

½ tsp of baking soda

½ tsp of cinnamon

½ tsp of nutmeg

1 medium avocado, sliced

2 large eggs

1½ tsp of vanilla, minced

1 tbsp. of coconut oil

½ cup of almond milk

Preparation:

Preheat the oven to 300°F.

In a large bowl, combine almond flour, coconut flour, baking soda, cinnamon, and nutmeg.

In another bowl, combine eggs, avocado slices, coconut oil and almond milk. Pour this mixture into a blender and mix well for about 30 seconds. Now combine these two mixtures using an electric mixer.

Pour into muffin molds and bake for about 20 minutes. Remove from the oven and allow it to cool for a while.

Nutrition information per serving: Kcal: 75, Protein: 4.5g, Carbs: 5.3g, Fats: 4.1g

30. Scrambled Eggs with Chopped Mint

Ingredients:

2 large eggs

1 tbsp. of olive oil

1 tbsp. of mint, finely chopped

1 cup of cherry tomatoes, chopped

1 small onion, diced

¼ tsp of black pepper, ground

Preparation:

Preheat the oil in a large saucepan over a medium-high temperature. Add chopped vegetables and reduce to low. Cook for about 15 minutes, or until liquid evaporates.

Beat the eggs and add chopped mint. Mix with vegetables and cook for 5 minutes. Add some pepper to taste before serving.

Nutrition information per serving: Kcal: 271, Protein: 13.6g, Carbs: 12.6g, Fats: 24.1g

31.   Mixed Berries Pancakes

Ingredients:

3 large eggs

½ cup of coconut flour

½ cup of almond flour

1 cup of coconut milk

1 tsp of apple vinegar

1 tsp vanilla, minced

½ tsp of baking soda

¼ tsp of salt

1 tsp of coconut oil

3 cups of fresh berries, mixed

Preparation:

Combine the coconut flour, almond flour, vanilla, baking soda, and salt in a large bowl. In a smaller bowl, mix coconut milk and apple vinegar. Whisk in the coconut mixture until smooth dough.

Using a nonstick skillet, heat up the coconut oil over a medium heat. Spread the desired amount of dough over the skillet. Use a spoon to smooth the surface of each pancake. Fry for about 2-3 minutes on each side.

Top with mixed fresh berries and 1 tbsp. of agave syrup.

Nutrition information per serving: Kcal: 173, Protein: 8.2g, Carbs: 22.1g, Fats: 13.2g

32.   Gluten-Free Burgers

Ingredients:

2 lbs. of ground beef

3 large eggs

2 medium-sized onions, peeled and sliced

2 tsp of coconut oil

½ cup of fresh tomato sauce

1 tsp of red pepper, minced

½ tsp of ground black pepper

Preparation:

Preheat the oven to 300°F.

Meanwhile, melt 2 teaspoons of coconut oil over a medium temperature in a nonstick skillet. Add onion slices and fry until translucent. Stir constantly. Remove from the skillet and set aside. Allow it to cool before combining with the meat.

In a large bowl, combine the meat with other ingredients. Mix well to evenly distribute the ingredients. Divide the mixture into 5 pieces and shape the burgers.

Bake for about 30 minutes, or until the meat is done. Remove from the oven and serve with lettuce, tomato, or some other vegetables of your choice.

Nutrition information per serving: Kcal: 319, Protein: 47.4g, Carbs: 12.3g, Fats: 34.2g

33. Greek Pepper Salad

Ingredients:

½ red onion, peeled and sliced

½ cucumber, sliced

½ bell pepper, sliced

2 tbsp. of Greek yogurt

1 tbsp. of fresh parsley, finely chopped

5 tbsp. of extra virgin olive oil

Pepper to taste

Salt to taste

Preparation:

Combine the Greek yogurt with fresh parsley. Add some salt and pepper and mix well.

Slice the vegetables and arrange on a serving platter. Add a generous amount of olive oil and top with Greek yogurt mixture. Serve immediately.

Nutrition information per serving: Kcal: 118, Protein: 16g, Carbs: 29g, Fats: 21g

34.   Mushroom Omelet

Ingredients:

1 cup of button mushrooms, sliced

2 large eggs

1 tsp of fresh rosemary, chopped

¼ tsp of dry oregano

1 tbsp. of olive oil

Preparation:

Heat up the olive oil in a large skillet, over a medium temperature. Add button mushrooms and cook for 3-4 minutes, until the water evaporates. Remove from the skillet.

In a small bowl, whisk together eggs, rosemary and oregano. Pour the mixture in the skillet and fry for about 4 minutes. When eggs are set, layer half of the skillet with mushrooms. Fold untopped half of the omelet over filling and fry for one more minute. Move to a plate and serve with few lettuce leaves, but this is optional.

Nutritional information per serving: Kcal: 195, Protein: 16g, Carbs: 1.4g, Fats: 21g

35. Papaya Flaxseeds Smoothie

Ingredients:

1 medium-sized papaya, chopped

1 tsp of flaxseed, ground

1 cup of plain yogurt, fat-free

½ cup of pineapple, chopped

1 tsp of coconut extract

Preparation:

Combine all ingredients in a food processor. Blend until smooth and transfer to a serving glasses. Add some crushed ice and serve.

Nutrition information per serving: Kcal: 298, Protein: 12.4g, Carbs: 64.5g, Fats: 1.5g

36.   Coco Pancakes

Ingredients:

1 cup of coconut flour

1 tbsp. of baking soda

2 free-range eggs

1 cup of coconut milk

½ cup of water

¼ tsp of sea salt

¼ tsp of cinnamon

1 tbsp. of coconut oil

Preparation:

Combine all dry ingredients with coconut milk and water. Mix well to make a smooth dough. Add some cinnamon to taste and fry over a medium heat for about 3-4 minutes on each side. These pancakes are perfect with strawberries on top.

Nutritional information per serving: Kcal: 371, Protein: 35g, Carbs: 41g, Fats: 23g

37. Almond Flour Muffins

Ingredients:

1 cup of almond flour

¼ cup of coconut flour

¼ tsp of baking soda

½ cup of coconut milk

2 tbsp. of coconut oil

2 free-range eggs

½ cup of fresh raspberries

Preparation:

Preheat the oven to 300°F.

In a large bowl, combine all dry ingredients and mix well. In a separate bowl, whisk together coconut milk, coconut oil, and eggs. Gently combine these two mixtures and add raspberries. Spread the mixture into muffin molds and bake for about 20 minutes.

Nutritional information per serving: Kcal: 120, Protein: 3g, Carbs: 18.9g, Fats: 12g

38.   Banana Toast

Ingredients:

1 cup of almond flour

1 tsp of baking soda

2 large bananas, sliced

1 cup of Brazil nuts, minced

2 tbsp. of coconut oil

2 large eggs

1 tsp of vanilla extract, sugar-free

½ tsp of cinnamon

For the filling:

2 large eggs

⅓ cup of coconut milk

1 tsp of vanilla extract, sugar-free

¼ teaspoon of cinnamon

1 tbsp. of coconut oil

Preparation:

Preheat oven to 350°F.

Using an electric mixer, combine the Brazil nuts and coconut oil until you get a smooth butter mixture.

Peel the bananas and chop them roughly. Add coconut mixture and banana slices in a food processor and combine for about a minute.

Combine almond flour, baking soda, vanilla extract and cinnamon in a large bowl. Whisk in eggs and banana mixture and make a smooth dough.

Spread the dough over a small baking sheet (the size depends on how thick you want your bread to be). Place in the oven and bake for about 25 minutes, or until light brown color. Remove from the oven and allow it to cool for a while.

Cut the bread into 1-inch slices. Set aside.

In a smaller bowl, combine the eggs, coconut milk, vanilla extract and cinnamon. Use a large, nonstick skillet to heat up 1 tbsp. of coconut oil, over a medium temperature. Dip the bread slices in your egg mixture and fry for about 2 minutes on each side. Use a kitchen paper to remove the excess oil and serve.

Nutritional information per serving: Kcal: 180, Protein: 16g, Carbs: 28g, Fats: 10g

39.   Baked Sweet Potatoes

Ingredients:

2 medium-sized sweet potatoes, peeled and halved

1 chicken breast, boneless and skinless

3 free-range eggs

1/4 cup of whole milk

1 tbsp. of olive oil

Preparation:

Preheat the oven to 350°F.

Wash and peel the potatoes. Cut each potato in half and bake for about 50 minutes. Remove from the oven and let it stand for about 10 minutes.

Now, scoop out the middle of each potato and set aside.

Heat up the olive oil in a medium-sized skillet. Fry the chicken breast for few minutes and remove from the skillet. Chop into small pieces.

In a separate bowl, whisk eggs and milk. Add scooped parts of sweet potatoes and mix well. Combine this mixture with chopped chicken sausage and fill each potato half with this mixture. Put it back in the oven and bake for 15 more minutes.

Remove from the oven and chill.

40. Blueberry Green Tea Smoothie

Ingredients:

1 cup of blueberries, frozen

1 green tea bag

½ cup of vanilla yogurt

1 medium-sized banana, sliced

2 tbsp. of honey

4 tbsp. of water

Preparation:

Heat up the water in small pot until steaming hot. Remove from the heat and put green tea bag inside. Let it stand for 3-4 minutes. now, add honey and stir until melts.

Combine blueberries, yogurt, and banana in a food processor. Add previously prepared tea and honey and blend until smooth. If the mixture is too thick, add some water. Transfer to a serving glasses.

Serve cold.

Nutrition information per serving: Kcal: 269, Protein: 3.2g, Carbs: 51.5g, Fats: 2.6g

41.   Greek Yogurt Chicken

Ingredients:

1 lb. of chicken thighs, skinless, boneless, and chopped

6 oz. of Greek yogurt

2 garlic cloves, crushed

1 tbsp. of lemon juice

1 tsp of lemon zest

1 tsp of salt

1 tsp of dried oregano, ground

¼ tsp of black pepper, ground

Preparation:

Combine chicken, Greek yogurt, garlic, salt, and pepper in a slow cooker. Add water if too thick. Seal the lid and cook for 6-7 hours. Remove from the heat and set aside for 30 minutes.

Transfer to the serving plate and drizzle with lemon juice. Sprinkle with oregano, salt, and pepper if needed and top with a pinch of a lemon zest.

Nutritional information per serving: Kcal: 311, Protein: 36g, Carbs: 30g, Fats: 27.5g

42.   Cheddar Broccoli Bake

Ingredients:

4 cups of fresh broccoli, chopped

½ cup of red onion, finely chopped

6 large eggs

1 cup of skim milk

1 cup of Cheddar cheese, shredded

2 tbsp. of fresh water

½ tsp of salt

½ tsp of black pepper, ground

Preparation:

Preheat the oven to 350°F.

Place broccoli and onion in a large saucepan over a medium-high temperature. Add 2 tablespoons of water and cook for about 7-8 minutes, or until soft and tender. Remove from the heat and drain the excessive liquid. Set aside.

Combine eggs, milk, and cheese in a large mixing bowl and whisk well to combine. Add the broccoli mixture and a pinch of black pepper. Toss well to combine.

Take a large baking dish and spread the mixture evenly. Bake for about 30 minutes. It is done if the fork is clean after inserted. Remove from the heat and top with some extra shredded cheese if you like. Let it cool for a while and serve.

Nutritional information per serving: Kcal: 298, Protein: 36g, Carbs: 42.5g, Fats: 27g

43.   Blueberry Grape Pudding

Ingredients:

8 oz. of blueberries, frozen

8 oz. of fresh black grapes

2 large eggs

2 tbsp. of almonds, chopped

2 tbsp. of cashews, chopped

2 tbsp. of honey

1 tsp of lemon zest

1 tbsp. of cornstarch

1 tsp of cinnamon, ground

½ cup of water

Preparation:

Combine all ingredients except cornstarch in a large pot. Cover with a lid and cook for 2 hours on a medium temperature.

Meanwhile, combine cornstarch with a tablespoon of water and mix well. Pour the mixture into the pot and continue to cook for 45 minutes. Remove from the heat and let it cool completely.

Transfer to the serving bowl and refrigerate for 1 hour. Sprinkle with cinnamon before serving.

Nutritional information per serving: Kcal: 190, Protein: 1.9g, Carbs: 17g, Fats: 6g

44. Ginger Smoothie

Ingredients:

½ tsp of fresh ginger, grated

1 large banana, sliced

6 oz. of vanilla yogurt

1 tbsp. of honey, raw

Preparation:

Combine all ingredients in a blender. Blend until smooth and transfer to a serving glass. Refrigerate 30 minutes before serving.

Nutrition information per serving: Kcal: 157, Protein: 4.8g, Carbs: 34.2g, Fats: 1.3g

45.   Chicken Apricot Burgers with Mustard

Ingredients:

1 lb. of chicken breasts, shredded

1 medium-sized onion, sliced

2 garlic cloves, minced

3 tbsp. of yellow mustard

1 cup of apricots, chopped

1 tsp of apple cider vinegar

½ tsp of salt

½ cup of fresh basil, chopped

½ tsp of black pepper, ground

2 burger buns, multi-grain

Preparation:

Combine meat, onion, garlic, mustard, apricots, vinegar, basil, salt, and pepper in a slow cooker. Add enough water to cover all ingredients. Seal the lid and cook for 6 hours. Remove from the heat and let it cool for a while.

Form the burgers using hands and place into buns. Use a toothpick to secure the burgers. You can use some more fresh vegetables for some extra taste and nutrients.

Nutritional information per serving: Kcal: 396, Protein: 35g, Carbs: 31.6g, Fats: 19g

46.   Quinoa and Raisins Breakfast Cereal

Ingredients:

1 cup of white quinoa, pre-cooked

1 tbsp. of raisins

1 tbsp. of almonds, chopped

1 tsp of chia seeds

¼ tsp of cinnamon

1 cup of water

1 tbsp. of honey

Preparation:

Combine quinoa, raisins, almonds and chia into a mixing bowl. Stir well to combine.

Bring one cup of water to boil and pour it into the bowl. Give it a good stir. Cover and set aside for 10 minutes.

If the water is absorbed, add honey and stir well once again. Transfer to a serving bowl.

Nutrition information per serving: Kcal: 211, Protein: 6.2g, Carbs: 29.8g, Fats: 8.1g

47.   Seeds and Strawberry Smoothie

Ingredients:

1 tbsp. of flaxseed oil, organic

1 tbsp. of pumpkin seeds

1 cup of frozen strawberries, unsweetened

1 cup of skim milk

Preparation:

Combine milk and strawberries in a blender. Blend for 1 minute or until smooth. Transfer to a serving glass and stir in, or top with seeds.

Refrigerate 20 minutes before serving.

Nutrition information per serving: Kcal: 256, Protein: 9.2g, Carbs: 26.7g, Fats: 14.3g

48.   Romaine Salad

Ingredients:

6 cups of Romaine lettuce, chopped

2 tbsp. of feta cheese, crumbled

¼ cup of dried cherries, chopped

1 tbsp. of shallots, minced

2 tbsp. of extra-virgin olive oil

2 tbsp. of balsamic vinegar

1 tbsp. of fresh parsley, finely chopped

1 tbsp. of Dijon mustard

¼ tsp of salt

1 garlic clove, crushed

¼ tsp of black pepper, ground

Preparation:

Combine oil, vinegar, garlic, parsley, shallots, mustard, salt, and pepper in a small mixing bowl. Stir well to combine and set aside to allow the flavors to mingle.

Now, combine lettuce, cherries, and cheese in serving bowl. Drizzle with dressing and give it a good stir to combine.

Serve.

Nutrition information per serving: Kcal: 131, Protein: 1.9g, Carbs: 13.7g, Fats: 8.5g

49.   Strawberry Honey Smoothie

Ingredients:

2 large bananas

10oz strawberries, halved

2 small green apples, cored

2 tbsp. raw honey

2 cups of coconut milk

Preparation:

Place the ingredients in a blender and pulse to combine. Serve immediately.

Nutritional information per serving: Kcal: 145, Protein: 7g, Carbs: 31g, Fats: 2.1g

50.   Kidney Bean Salad

Ingredients:

1 whole egg, boiled

1 cup of lettuce, finely chopped

½ cup of green beans, cooked

½ cup kidney beans, cooked

4 cherry tomatoes, halved

Few black olives, sliced

3 tbsp. of extra virgin olive oil

½ tsp of salt

1 tbsp. of fresh lemon juice

Preparation:

First you want to boil the egg. Gently place the egg into a pot with just enough water to cover. Bring to a boil and cook for 10 minutes. You can use a kitchen timer. After 10 minutes, drain the water and place the egg under the cold water. Peel and slice

Meanwhile, combine other ingredients in a large bowl. Add the olive oil, fresh lemon juice, and salt. Toss well to combine. Top with sliced eggs and serve.

To prevent the ingredients from changing the color in leftover salad, cover tightly with a plastic wrap. Keep in the refrigerator.

Nutritional information per serving: Kcal: 270, Protein: 19g, Carbs: 44g, Fats: 18g

51. Wild Berries with Nutmeg

Ingredients:

1cup of mixed fresh berries

5-6 medium-sized strawberries

½ pear, sliced

2oz fresh spinach

¼ fresh orange juice

1 tsp of sugar

¼ tsp of nutmeg

Preparation:

In a small bowl, combine the fresh orange juice with sugar and nutmeg. Mix well with a fork.

Wash and gently rinse the spinach. You don't want to squeeze it as this will take away a lot of great nutrients. Place on a serving plate.

Wash and pat dry the pear. Slice and make another layer on your plate. Top with mixed berries and orange juice dressing. Serve cold.

A great tip is to leave it in the freezer for just ten minutes before serving.

Nutritional information per serving: Kcal: 136, Protein: 0.2g, Carbs: 29g, Fats: 0.3g

52. Spring Chicken Breast

Ingredients:

½ piece of chicken breast, boneless and skinless

4 lettuce leaves, rinsed

½ cucumber, sliced

½ red bell pepper, sliced

Few black olives, pitted

3 tbsp. of olive oil

½ tsp of salt

½ tsp of ground turmeric

Preparation:

Wash and pat dry the meat using a kitchen paper. Slice into 0.5-inch-thick slices. Heat up a non-stick frying pan over a medium temperature. Add the chicken fillets and fry for about 4 minutes on each side. You can add some water if necessary (2-3 tablespoons at a time will be enough). Remove from the heat and set aside.

Place the lettuce leaves on a serving platter. Make another layer with sliced cucumber and sliced bell peppers. Add olives and top with chicken. Season with olive oil, salt, and ground turmeric.

Nutritional information per serving: Kcal: 274, Protein: 24g, Carbs: 30g, Fats: 16.5g

53.   Creamy Sweet Corn Salad

Ingredients:

½ cup of lettuce, finely chopped

½ ripe tomato, sliced

2 tbsp. of sweet corn

Few black olives, pitted

½ cup of Greek yogurt

¼ cup of fresh parsley, finely chopped

2 tbsp. of olive oil

½ tsp of salt

½ tsp of ground black pepper

Preparation:
In a small bowl, combine the Greek yogurt with finely chopped parsley, olive oil, salt, and ground black pepper. Mix well with an electric mixer, until smooth mixture.

Combine the vegetables and top with Greek yogurt mixture. Serve cold.

Nutritional information per serving: Kcal: 123, Protein: 16g, Carbs: 41g, Fats: 17g

54.   Shrimp Veggie Skewers

Ingredients:

1 small tomato, chopped into bite-sized pieces

¼ cucumber, sliced

1lb shrimps, peeled

3 black olives

2 lettuce leaves, chopped

½ cup of olive oil

¼ cup of fresh lime juice

½ tsp of sea salt

Preparation:

Shake together olive oil, fresh lime juice, and sea salt. Place the ingredients in this mixture and let it stand for about 30 minutes.

Place three wooden skewers into a large pot with some water to soak. This little trick will prevent the skewers from burning. Remove the ingredients from the marinade and divide between the skewers. Grill for about 3-4 minutes. Serve immediately.

Nutritional information per serving: Kcal: 123, Protein: 16g, Carbs: 41g, Fats: 17g

55.   Almond Spinach Smoothie

Ingredients:

1 cup of spinach, chopped

¼ of cucumber, peeled and sliced

1 tbsp. of celery, finely chopped

1 tbsp. of flaxseeds

¼ cup of strawberries, frozen

1 tsp of cinnamon, ground

6oz of almond milk

Preparation:

Combine the ingredients in a blender and mix well for 20-30 seconds, or until smooth.

Serve cold.

Nutritional information per serving: Kcal: 164, Protein: 4.3g, Carbs: 31.4g, Fats: 3.7g

56.   Brown Lentil and Pasta Soup

Ingredients:

4 oz. lean turkey breast, cut into small squares

1 onion, chopped

2 garlic cloves, crushed

2 celery sticks, chopped

1¾ oz. spaghetti, broken into small pieces

14 oz. canned brown lentils, drained

2 pints' hot vegetable stock

2 tbsp. chopped fresh mint

Preparation:

Place the turkey in a large, dry frying pan together with the onions, garlic and celery. Cook for 4-5 minutes, stirring, until the onion is tender and the bacon is just beginning to brown.

Add the pasta to the frying pan and cook, stirring, for about 1 minute.

Add the brown lentils and stock and bring the mixture to a boil. Lower the heat and leave to simmer for about 12-15 minutes or until the pasta is tender.

Remove the frying pan from the heat and stir in the chopped fresh mint.

Transfer the soup to warm soup bowls and serve immediately.

Nutritional information per serving: Kcal: 225, Protein: 13g, Carbs: 27g, Fats: 8g

57. Creamy Asparagus Soup

Ingredients:

2 lb. of fresh asparagus, trimmed and chopped

2 medium-sized onions, chopped

1 cup of fresh celery, diced

2 tbsp. of butter, unsalted

1tbsp of fresh parsley, finely chopped

1 tbsp. of skim milk

4 cups of chicken broth

1 tbsp. of parmesan cheese, shredded

1 tsp of yellow mustard

1 tbsp. of lemon juice

1 tsp of salt

1 tsp of black pepper, ground

Preparation:

Melt the butter in a large pot over a medium-high temperature. Add the onions and celery and sauté until soften or translucent.

Add the asparagus, parsley, and lemon juice. Pour the broth over and bring it to a boil. Reduce the heat to low and simmer for 15 minutes. Remove from the heat.

Now, remove the asparagus from the pan and gently transfer to the food processor. Blend until smooth and return the mixture to the pot.

Stir in all other ingredients and cook for 5 minutes more on low temperature. Remove from the heat and serve warm.

Nutrition information per serving: Kcal: 161, Protein: 5.3g, Carbs: 18.3g, Fats: 8.5g

JUICES

1.   Blueberry Basil Juice

Ingredients:

1 cup of blueberries

1 cup of fresh basil, torn

1 cup of strawberries, sliced

1 whole lemon, peeled

1 small Granny Smith's apple, cored

Preparation:

Place the blueberries in a colander and rinse under cold running water. Slightly drain and set aside.

Wash the basil thoroughly and torn with hands. Set aside.

Wash the strawberries and remove the stems. Cut into slices and fill the measuring cup. Reserve the rest for later.

Peel the lemon and cut lengthwise in half. Set aside.

Wash the apple and cut in half. Remove the core and cut into bite-sized pieces. Set aside.

Now, combine blueberries, basil, strawberries, lemon, and apple in a juicer and process until juiced. Transfer to a serving glass and add few ice cubes.

Serve immediately.

Nutritional information per serving: Kcal: 193, Protein: 4.3g, Carbs: 60.1g, Fats: 1.6g

2.   Tomato Mustard Green Juice

Ingredients:

1 medium-sized Roma tomato, chopped

1 cup of mustard greens, torn

1 cup of fresh spinach, torn

1 large carrot, sliced

1 tsp of fresh rosemary, finely chopped

Preparation:

Wash the tomato and place it in a bowl. Cut into bite-sized pieces and make sure to reserve tomato juices while cutting. Set aside.

Wash mustard greens and spinach thoroughly under cold running water. Slightly drain and torn with hands. Set aside.

Wash and peel the carrot. Cut into thin slices and set aside.

Now, combine tomato, mustard greens, spinach, carrot, and rosemary in a juicer and process until juiced. Transfer to a serving glass and stir in the reserved tomato juice. Refrigerate for 15 minutes before serving.

Enjoy!

Nutritional information per serving: Kcal: 74, Protein: 9.4g, Carbs: 21.9g, Fats: 1.5g

3.   Watercress Celery Juice

Ingredients:

2 cups of fresh watercress, chopped

2 large celery stalks, chopped

1 cup of cucumber, sliced

1 whole lime, peeled

¼ tsp of turmeric, ground

1 oz of water

Preparation:

Place the watercress in a large colander. Rinse under cold running water. Torn with hands and set aside.

Wash the celery stalks and cut into bite-sized pieces. Set aside.

Wash the cucumber and cut into thin slices. Fill the measuring cup and reserve the rest for later.

Peel the lime and cut lengthwise in half. Set aside.

Now, combine watercress, celery, cucumber, and lime in a juicer. Process until juiced. Transfer to a serving glass and stir in the turmeric and water.

Refrigerate for 10 minutes before serving.

Enjoy!

Nutritional information per serving: Kcal: 35, Protein: 2.9g, Carbs: 10.3g, Fats: 0.4g

4.   Orange Carrot Juice

Ingredients:

1 large orange, peeled

1 small carrot, sliced

1 small banana, sliced

2 whole plums, chopped

Preparation:

Peel the orange and divide into wedges. Cut each wedge in half and set aside.

Wash and peel the carrot. Cut into thin slices and set aside.

Peel the banana and cut into small chunks. Set aside.

Wash the plums and cut in half. Remove the pits and cut into bite-sized pieces. Set aside.

Now, combine orange, carrot, banana, and plums in a juicer and process until juiced. Transfer to a serving glass and add some ice before serving.

Nutritional information per serving: Kcal: 214, Protein: 4.2g, Carbs: 64.5g, Fats: 1.1g

5.   Grapefruit Beet Juice

Ingredients:

1 whole grapefruit, peeled

1 whole beet, chopped

1 small zucchini, chopped

1 cup of fresh basil, roughly chopped

1 tbsp of liquid honey

Preparation:

Peel the grapefruit and divide into wedges. Cut each wedge in half and set aside.

Wash and trim off the beet. Slightly peel and cut into bite-sized pieces. Set aside.

Peel the zucchini and chop into small chunks. Set aside.

Wash the basil thoroughly under cold running water. Slightly drain and roughly chop it. Set aside.

Now, combine grapefruit, beet, zucchini, and basil in a juicer and process until juiced. Transfer to a serving glass and stir in the honey.

Add some crushed ice before serving and enjoy!

Nutritional information per serving: Kcal: 192, Protein: 5.4g, Carbs: 38.4g, Fats: 1.1g

6. Broccoli Kale Juice

Ingredients:

2 cups of broccoli, chopped

2 cups of kale, roughly chopped

2 medium-sized asparagus spears, trimmed

1 cup of fresh mint, torn

1 whole lemon, peeled

1 small ginger knob, peeled

Preparation:

Trim off the outer leaves of the broccoli. Wash it and cut into bite-sized pieces. Set aside.

Rinse the kale under cold running water. Slightly drain and torn with hands. Set aside.

Wash the asparagus and trim off the woody ends. Cut into small pieces and set aside.

Wash the mint and roughly chop it. You can soak it in water for 5 minutes before preparation, but it's optional. Set aside.

Peel the ginger knob and set aside.

Peel the lemon and cut lengthwise in half. Set aside.

Now, combine broccoli, kale, asparagus, ginger, mint, and lemon in a juicer. Process until juiced. Transfer to a serving glass and refrigerate for 15 minutes before serving.

Nutritional information per serving: Kcal: 118, Protein: 13.3g, Carbs: 35.3g, Fats: 2.4g

7.   Cranberry Kiwi Juice

Ingredients:

1 cup of cranberries, chopped

1 whole kiwi, peeled

1 small Granny Smith's apple, cored

1 small orange, peeled

¼ tsp of cinnamon, ground

Preparation:

Wash the cranberries and place them in a bowl. Chop into small pieces and set aside.

Peel the kiwi and cut into bite-sized pieces. Set aside.

Wash the apple and cut in half. Remove the core and cut into small pieces. Set aside.

Peel the orange and divide into wedges. Cut each wedge in half and set aside.

Now, combine cranberries, kiwi, apple, and orange in a juicer. Process until juiced.

Transfer to a serving glass and stir in the cinnamon. Add some crushed ice and serve immediately.

Nutritional information per serving: Kcal: 183, Protein: 3.1g, Carbs: 58.5g, Fats: 0.9g

8.   Watermelon Guava Juice

Ingredients:

1 cup of watermelon, chopped

1 whole guava, chunked

1 cup of pomegranate seeds

1 cup of cucumber, sliced

1 tbsp of liquid honey

Preparation:

Cut the watermelon lengthwise. For one cup, you will need a large slice. Peel and cut into small pieces. Remove the seeds and set aside. Reserve the rest for some other juices.

Peel the guava and cut into small chunks. Set aside.

Cut the top of the pomegranate fruit using a sharp paring knife. Slice down to each of the white membranes inside of the fruit. Pop the seeds into a measuring cup and set aside.

Wash the cucumber and cut into thin slices. Fill the measuring cup and reserve the rest in the refrigerator. Set aside.

Now, combine watermelon, guava, pomegranate, and cucumber in a juicer and process until juiced. Transfer to a serving glass and stir in the honey.

Add some ice and serve immediately.

Nutritional information per serving: Kcal: 134, Protein: 4.1g, Carbs: 37.5g, Fats: 1.8g

9.   Cherry Mango Juice

Ingredients:

1 cup of organic cherries, pitted

1 cup of mango, chunked

1 cup of fresh spinach, roughly chopped

1 cup of mustard greens, chopped

Preparation:

Wash the cherries and remove the stems. Cut each cherry in half and remove the pits. Fill the measuring cup and reserve the rest for later.

Peel the mango and cut into small chunks. Fill the measuring cup and reserve the rest for later.

Combine spinach and mustard greens in a large colander. Rinse thoroughly under cold water. Slightly drain and roughly chop it. Set aside.

Now, combine cherries, mango, spinach, and mustard greens in a juicer and process until juiced. Transfer to a serving glass and refrigerate for 10 minutes before serving.

Enjoy!

Nutritional information per serving: Kcal: 209, Protein: 10.6g, Carbs: 59.6g, Fats: 2.1g

10.   Zucchini Lemon Juice

Ingredients:

1 small zucchini, chopped

1 whole lemon, peeled

1 medium-sized carrot, sliced

1 cup of green grapes

1 tbsp of liquid honey

Preparation:

Wash the zucchini and cut into bite-sized pieces. Set aside.

Peel the lemon and cut lengthwise in half. Set aside.

Wash the carrot and slightly peel it. Cut into thin slices and set aside.

Wash the grapes and fill the measuring cup. Set aside.

Now, combine zucchini lemon, carrot, and grapes in a juicer and process until juiced. Transfer to a serving glass and stir in the honey.

Refrigerate for 15 minutes before serving.

Enjoy!

Nutritional information per serving: Kcal: 163, Protein: 3.2g, Carbs: 37.7g, Fats: 1.1g

11.   Artichoke Basil Juice

Ingredients:

1 medium-sized artichoke, chopped

1 cup of fresh basil, torn

1 cup of sweet potatoes, cubed

1 small green apple, cored

Preparation:

Trim off the outer leaves of the artichoke using a sharp paring knife. Wash it and cut into bite-sized pieces. Set aside.

Wash the basil thoroughly under cold running water. Slightly drain and roughly chop it. Set aside.

Peel the sweet potatoes and cut into small cubes. Fill the measuring cup and reserve the rest for later. Set aside.

Wash the apple and cut in half. Remove the core and cut into bite-sized pieces. Set aside.

Now, combine artichoke, basil, potatoes, and apple in a juicer. Process until juiced and transfer to a serving glass.

Stir in the turmeric and serve immediately.

Nutritional information per serving: Kcal: 202, Protein: 7.6g, Carbs: 60.4g, Fats: 0.7g

12.   Pepper Broccoli Juice

Ingredients:

1 large red bell pepper, chopped

1 cup of broccoli, chopped

1 cup of Brussels sprouts, halved

1 cup of Romaine lettuce, shredded

1 cup of Swiss chard, torn

Preparation:

Wash the bell pepper and cut in half. Remove the seeds and chop into small pieces. Set aside.

Wash the broccoli and trim off the outer leaves. Cut into bite-sized pieces and fill the measuring cup. Reserve the rest for later. Set aside.

Wash the Brussels sprouts and trim off the outer wilted layers. Cut each in half and set aside.

Combine lettuce and Swiss chard in a colander. Rinse thoroughly under cold running water. Torn with hands and set aside.

Now, combine bell pepper, broccoli, Brussels sprouts, lettuce, and Swiss chard in a juicer and process until juiced. Transfer to a serving glass and refrigerate for about 10-15 minutes before serving.

You can stir in some turmeric for some extra taste. However, it's optional.

Nutritional information per serving: Kcal: 92, Protein: 8.4g, Carbs: 26.7g, Fats: 1.3g

13. Cauliflower Avocado Juice

Ingredients:

5 cauliflower flowerets, chopped

1 cup of avocado, cubed

1 whole lime, peeled

1 whole leek, chopped

Preparation:

Wash the cauliflower flowerets thoroughly and chop into small pieces. Set aside.

Peel the avocado and cut in half. Remove the pit and cut into small cubes. Fill the measuring cup and reserve the rest in the refrigerator. Set aside.

Peel the lime and cut lengthwise in half. Set aside.

Wash the leek and cut into small pieces. Set aside.

Now, combine cauliflower, avocado, lime, and leek in a juicer and process until juiced. Transfer to a serving glass and refrigerate for 10 minutes before serving.

Enjoy!

Nutritional information per serving: Kcal: 268, Protein: 5.7g, Carbs: 32.4g, Fats: 22.5g

14. Kale Cucumber Juice

Ingredients:

2 cups of fresh kale, chopped

1 cup of cucumber, sliced

1 medium-sized green bell pepper, chopped

1 cup of watercress, torn

1 cup of fresh parsley, torn

1 oz of water

Preparation:

Wash the kale thoroughly under cold running water. Chop into small pieces and set aside.

Wash the cucumber and cut into thin slices. Fill the measuring cup and reserve the rest for later. Set aside.

Wash the bell pepper and cut in half. Remove the seeds and chop into small pieces. Set aside.

Combine watercress and parsley in a colander. Rinse well under cold running water and torn with hands. Set aside.

Now, combine kale, cucumber, bell pepper, watercress, and parsley in a juicer and process until juiced. Transfer to a serving glass and stir in the water. Add some ice before serving.

Enjoy!

Nutritional information per serving: Kcal: 86, Protein: 9.6g, Carbs: 23.4g, Fats: 2g

15.   Strawberry Lemon Juice

Ingredients:

10 large strawberries, chopped

1 whole lemon, peeled

1 cup of raspberries

1 small green apple, cored

¼ tsp of cinnamon, ground

Preparation:

Wash the strawberries and remove the stems. Cut into small pieces and set aside.

Peel the lemon and cut lengthwise in half. Set aside.

Wash the raspberries using a colander. Rinse under cold water and slightly drain. Set aside.

Wash the apple and cut in half. Remove the core and cut into bite-sized pieces. Set aside.

Now, combine strawberries, lemon, raspberries, and apple in a juicer and process until juiced. Transfer to a serving glass and stir in the cinnamon.

Add some ice and serve immediately.

Nutritional information per serving: Kcal: 151, Protein: 3.9g, Carbs: 53.5g, Fats: 3.9g

16.   Blackberry Beet Juice

Ingredients:

1 cup of fresh blackberries

1 cup of beets, trimmed

1 whole lime, peeled

1 medium-sized orange, peeled

Preparation:

Wash the blackberries thoroughly under cold running water. Slightly drain and set aside.

Wash the beets and trim off the green parts. Slightly peel and cut into thin slices. Fill the measuring cup and reserve the rest for later. You can keep the greens for some other juice.

Peel the lime and cut lengthwise in half. Set aside.

Peel the orange and divide into wedges. Cut each wedge in half and set aside.

Now, combine blackberries, beets, lime, and orange in a juicer and process until juiced. Transfer to a serving glass and add some crushed ice.

Enjoy!

Nutritional information per serving: Kcal: 135, Protein: 5.6g, Carbs: 45.9g, Fats: 1.1g

17.   Squash Cabbage Juice

Ingredients:

1 cup of butternut squash, chopped

1 cup of purple cabbage, chopped

1 large carrot, sliced

1 cup of fresh basil leaves, torn

1 oz of water

Preparation:

Peel the squash and cut in half. Scoop out the seeds and cut one large wedge. Cut into bite-sized pieces and fill the measuring cup. Wrap the rest in a plastic foil and store in the refrigerator for later.

Wash the cabbage and chop into small pieces. Fill the measuring cup and set aside.

Wash and peel the carrot. Cut into thin slices and set aside.

Rinse the basil leaves under cold running water. Roughly chop it and set aside.

Now, combine squash, cabbage, carrot, and basil in a juicer and process until juiced. Transfer to a serving glass and stir in the water. You can add a pinch of salt or red pepper if you like, but it's optional.

Serve immediately.

Nutritional information per serving: Kcal: 98, Protein: 4.1g, Carbs: 30.5g, Fats: 0.6g

18.   Tomato Parsley Juice

Ingredients:

1 cup of cherry tomatoes, halved

1 cup of fresh parsley, chopped

1 cup of cucumber, sliced

1 large red bell pepper, chopped

1 slice of onion

¼ tsp of salt

Preparation:

Wash the cherry tomatoes and remove the stems. Cut each tomato in half and set aside.

Wash the parsley thoroughly and torn with hands. Set aside.

Wash the cucumber and cut into thin slices. Fill the measuring cup and reserve the rest for later. Set aside.

Wash the bell pepper and cut in half. Remove the seeds and cut into small pieces. Set aside.

Soak onion slice in salted water for 5 minutes to reduce the bitterness.

Now, combine tomatoes, parsley, cucumber, bell pepper, and onion in a juicer and process until juiced. Transfer to a serving glass and stir in the salt.

Enjoy!

Nutritional information per serving: Kcal: 73, Protein: 4.6g, Carbs: 20.2g, Fats: 1.2g

19. Apricot Cherry Juice

Ingredients:

2 whole apricots, pitted

1 cup of cherries, pitted

1 whole lemon, peeled

1 cup of fresh mint, chopped

1 small red apple, cored

Preparation:

Wash the apricots and cut in half. Remove the pits and chop into bite-sized pieces. Set aside.

Wash the cherries using a colander. Cut each cherry in half and remove the pits and set aside.

Peel the lemon and cut lengthwise in half. Set aside.

Wash the mint thoroughly and slightly drain. Roughly chop it and set aside.

Wash the apple and cut in half. Remove the core and cut into small pieces. Set aside.

Now, combine apricots, cherries, lemon, mint, and apple in a juicer and process until well juiced. Transfer to a serving glass and add few ice cubes before serving.

Enjoy!

Nutritional information per serving: Kcal: 195, Protein: 4.5g, Carbs: 59.1g, Fats: 1.1g

20.   Sweet Potato Apple Juice

Ingredients:

1 cup of sweet potatoes, cubed

1 small Granny Smith's apple, cored

1 cup of beet greens, chopped

1 cup of mustard greens, chopped

1 large yellow bell pepper, chopped

Preparation:

Peel the sweet potato and cut into small cubes. Fill the measuring cup and reserve the rest for later.

Wash the apple and cut in half. Remove the core and cut into bite-sized pieces. Set aside.

Combine beet greens and mustard greens in a colander. Wash under cold running water and slightly drain. Roughly chop it and set aside.

Wash the bell pepper and cut in half. Remove the seeds and cut into small pieces. Set aside.

Now, combine potatoes, apple, beet greens, mustard greens, and pepper in a juicer and process until juiced. Transfer to a serving glass and serve immediately.

You can add a pinch of salt, but it's optional.

Nutritional information per serving: Kcal: 219, Protein: 7.1g, Carbs: 62.4g, Fats: 1.1g

21.   Blueberry Guava Juice

Ingredients:

1 cup of blueberries

1 whole guava, chopped

1 large orange, peeled

1 cup of fresh mint, torn

1 small ginger knob

1 oz of coconut water

Preparation:

Wash the blueberries thoroughly using a colander. Set aside.

Peel the guava and chop into small pieces. Set aside.

Peel the orange and divide into wedges. Cut each wedge in half and set aside.

Wash the mint thoroughly and slightly drain. Set aside.

Now, combine blueberries, guava, orange, mint, and ginger in a juicer and process until well juiced. Transfer to a serving glass and stir in the coconut water.

Enjoy!

Nutritional information per serving: Kcal: 178, Protein: 5.3g, Carbs: 55.7g, Fats: 1.5g

22.   Avocado Mango Juice

Ingredients:

1 cup of avocado, cubed

1 cup of mango, chopped

1 medium-sized carrot, sliced

1 cup of cucumber, sliced

1 whole lime, peeled

Preparation:

Peel the avocado and cut in half. Remove the pit and cut into bite-sized pieces. Fill the measuring cup and reserve the rest for later. Set aside.

Peel the mango and cut into small chunks. Fill the measuring cup and reserve the rest in the refrigerator. Set aside.

Wash and peel the carrot. Cut into thin slices and set aside.

Wash the cucumber and cut into thin slices. Fill the measuring cup and reserve the rest for later.

Peel the lime and cut lengthwise in half. Set aside.

Now, combine avocado, mango, carrot, cucumber, and lime in a juicer and process until well juiced.

Transfer to a serving glass and serve immediately.

Nutritional information per serving: Kcal: 324, Protein: 5.4g, Carbs: 48.9g, Fats: 22.8g

23.   **Pineapple Celery Juice**

Ingredients:

1 cup of pineapple, chunked

1 large celery stalk, chopped

1 whole kiwi, peeled

1 small peach, chopped

1 oz of coconut water

Preparation:

Cut the top of a pineapple and peel it using a sharp knife. Cut into small chunks and fill the measuring cup. Reserve the rest of the pineapple in a refrigerator.

Wash the celery and cut into bite-sized pieces. Set aside.

Peel the kiwi and cut lengthwise in half. Set aside.

Wash the peach and cut in half. Remove the pit and cut into small pieces. Set aside.

Now, combine pineapple, celery, kiwi, and peach in a juicer and process until well juiced. Transfer to a serving glass and stir in the coconut water.

Add some crushed ice and serve immediately.

Nutritional information per serving: Kcal: 156, Protein: 3.3g, Carbs: 46.1g, Fats: 0.9g

24.   Apple Cinnamon Juice

Ingredients:

1 medium-sized Granny Smith's apple, cored

¼ tsp of cinnamon, ground

1 cup of cucumber, sliced

1 cup of fresh mint, chopped

1 oz of water

Preparation:

Wash the apple and cut lengthwise in half. Remove the core and cut into bite-sized pieces. Set aside.

Wash the cucumber and cut into thin slices. Fill the measuring cup and reserve the rest for later. Set aside.

Wash the mint thoroughly under cold running water. Slightly drain and chop it. Set aside.

Now, combine apple, cucumber, mint, and cinnamon in a juicer. Process until well juiced. Transfer to a serving glass and stir in the water.

Add some ice and serve.

Nutritional information per serving: Kcal: 95, Protein: 2.1g, Carbs: 28.4g, Fats: 0.6g

25.   Mango Cantaloupe Juice

Ingredients:

1 cup of mango, chunked

1 medium-sized wedge of cantaloupe

2 whole cherries, pitted

2 medium-sized strawberries, chopped

1 oz of coconut water

Preparation:

Peel the mango and cut into small chunks. Fill the measuring cup and reserve the rest in the refrigerator. Set aside.

Cut the cantaloupe in half. Scoop out the seeds and cut the wedge. Peel it and cut into chunks. Reserve the rest of the cantaloupe in a refrigerator.

Wash the cherries and cut in half. Remove the pits and set aside.

Wash the strawberries and remove the stems. Cut into bite-sized pieces and set aside.

Now, combine mango, cantaloupe, cherries, and strawberries in a juicer and process until well juiced. Transfer to a serving glass and stir in the coconut water.

Add few ice cubes and serve immediately.

Nutritional information per serving: Kcal: 124, Protein: 2.3g, Carbs: 34.8g, Fats: 0.8g

26.   Lemon Grapefruit Juice

Ingredients:

1 whole lemon, peeled

1 whole grapefruit, wedged

1 medium-sized blood orange, peeled

1 medium-sized banana, chunked

¼ tsp of ginger, ground

Preparation:

Peel the lemon and cut lengthwise in half. Set aside.

Peel the grapefruit and orange. Divide into wedges and cut each wedge in half. Set aside.

Peel the banana and cut into chunks. Set aside.

Now, combine lemon, grapefruit, orange, and banana in a juicer. Process until well juiced. Transfer to a serving glass and stir in the ginger.

Refrigerate for 10 minutes before serving.

Nutritional information per serving: Kcal: 241, Protein: 5.1g, Carbs: 73.9g, Fats: 1.1g

27. Pepper Celery Juice

Ingredients:

1 large red bell pepper, chopped

1 medium-sized celery stalk, chopped

1 cup of green peas

1 cup of fresh spinach, torn

¼ tsp of salt

¼ tsp of red pepper, ground

Preparation:

Wash the bell pepper and cut lengthwise in half. Remove the seeds and chop into small pieces. Set aside.

Wash the celery stalk and cut into small pieces. Set aside.

Rinse the green peas using a colander. Place them in a bowl and soak in water for at least 30 minutes before using. You can also cook peas to soften. However, it's optional.

Wash the spinach thoroughly and slightly drain. Torn with hands and set aside.

Now, combine bell pepper, celery, peas, and spinach in a juicer and process until juiced. Transfer to a serving glass and stir in the salt and pepper.

Serve immediately.

Nutritional information per serving: Kcal: 160, Protein: 16.9g, Carbs: 40.8g, Fats: 2.1g

28.   Basil Lime Juice

Ingredients:

2 cups of fresh basil, chopped

1 whole lime, peeled

1 cup of mustard greens, chopped

1 cup of beet greens, chopped

1 whole cucumber, sliced

Preparation:

Combine basil, mustard greens, and beet greens in a large colander. Wash thoroughly under cold running water. Roughly chop it and soak in lukewarm water for 10 minutes.

Peel the lime and cut lengthwise in half. Set aside.

Wash the cucumber and cut into thin slices. Set aside.

Now, combine basil, lime, mustard greens, beet greens, and cucumber in a juicer and process until well juiced. Transfer to a serving glass and refrigerate for 20 minutes before serving.

Enjoy!

Nutritional information per serving: Kcal: 67, Protein: 6.1g, Carbs: 20.1g, Fats: 0.9g

29. Collard Greens Avocado Juice

Ingredients:

2 cups of collard greens, torn

1 cup of avocado, cubed

1 cup of beets, chopped

1 cup of watercress, torn

¼ tsp of balsamic vinegar

¼ tsp of salt

Preparation:

Wash the collard greens thoroughly under cold running water. Place them in a bowl and add 2 cups of boiling water. Let it soak for 10 minutes. Slightly drain and set aside.

Peel the avocado and cut in half. Remove the pit and cut into small cubes. Fill the measuring cup and reserve the rest in the refrigerator. Set aside.

Wash the beets and trim off the green ends. Peel and cut into small pieces. Set aside.

Wash the watercress and torn with hands. Set aside.

Now, combine collard greens, avocado, beets, and watercress in a juicer. Process until well juiced and transfer to a serving glass. Stir in the vinegar and salt for some extra taste.

Refrigerate for 10 minutes before serving.

Nutritional information per serving: Kcal: 258, Protein: 8.2g, Carbs: 30.2g, Fats: 22.7g

30. Asparagus Lemon Juice

Ingredients:

2 cups of asparagus, chopped

1 whole lemon, peeled

1 cup of cucumber, sliced

1 cup of fresh parsley, torn

Preparation:

Wash the asparagus and trim off the woody ends. Cut into small pieces and set aside.

Peel the lemon and cut lengthwise in half. Set aside.

Wash the cucumber and cut into thin slices. Fill the measuring cup and reserve the rest for later.

Wash the parsley thoroughly under cold running water and slightly drain. Torn with hands and set aside.

Now, combine asparagus, lemon, cucumber, and parsley in a juicer and process until well juiced. Transfer to a serving glass and refrigerate for 15 minutes before serving.

Enjoy!

Nutritional information per serving: Kcal: 64, Protein: 8,6g, Carbs: 21.5g, Fats: 1.1g

31.   Vanilla Blackberry Juice

Ingredients:

1 cup of blackberries

¼ tsp of vanilla extract

1 cup of pomegranate seeds

5 large strawberries, chopped

1 large banana, peeled

Preparation:

Place the blackberries in a colander and rinse under cold water. Slightly shake to drain and set aside.

Cut the top of the pomegranate fruit using a sharp paring knife. Slice down to each of the white membranes inside of the fruit. Pop the seeds into a measuring cup and set aside.

Wash the strawberries and remove the stems. Cut into small pieces and set aside.

Peel the banana and cut into small chunks. Set aside.

Now, combine blackberries, pomegranate, strawberries, banana, and vanilla extract in a juicer and process until juiced.

Transfer to a serving glass and add some crushed ice.

Serve immediately.

Nutritional information per serving: Kcal: 249, Protein: 7.5g, Carbs: 81.9g, Fats: 3.2g

32.   Avocado Mint Juice

Ingredients:

1 cup of avocado, chunked

1 cup of fresh mint, chopped

2 whole kiwis, peeled

3 whole plums, chopped

1 oz of water

Preparation:

Peel the avocado and cut lengthwise in half. Remove the pit and cut into small chunks. Fill the measuring cup and reserve the rest in the refrigerator. Set aside.

Wash the mint thoroughly under cold running water. Roughly chop it and set aside.

Peel the kiwis and cut lengthwise in half. Set aside.

Wash the plums and cut in half. Remove the pits and cut into bite-sized pieces. Set aside.

Now, combine avocado, mint, kiwis, and plums in a juicer and process until juiced. Transfer to a serving glass and stir in the water.

Refrigerate for 10 minutes before serving.

Enjoy!

Nutritional information per serving: Kcal: 356, Protein: 6.9g, Carbs: 59.4g, Fats: 23.5g

33.   Spinach Fennel Juice

Ingredients:

1 cup of fresh spinach, torn

1 cup of fennel, sliced

1 medium-sized celery stalk, chopped

1 medium-sized artichoke, chopped

Preparation:

Wash the spinach thoroughly under cold running water. Slightly drain and torn with hands. Set aside.

Wash the fennel bulb and trim off the wilted outer layers. Cut into small pieces and fill the measuring cup. Reserve the rest for some other juice.

Wash the celery stalk and cut into bite-sized pieces. Set aside.

Trim off the outer leaves of the artichoke using a sharp paring knife. Wash it and cut into bite-sized pieces. Set aside.

Now, combine spinach, fennel, celery, and artichoke in a juicer and process until well juiced. Transfer to a serving glass and refrigerate for 10 minutes before serving. You can add some salt to taste, but it's optional.

Nutritional information per serving: Kcal: 80, Protein: 11.5g, Carbs: 28.6g, Fats: 1.3g

34.   Papaya Mango Juice

Ingredients:

1 cup of papaya, chunked

1 cup of mango, chopped

1 whole apricot, chopped

1 small ginger knob, peeled

2 oz of coconut water

Preparation:

Peel the papaya and cut into small chunks. Fill the measuring cup and reserve the rest in the refrigerator. Set aside.

Peel the mango and cut into small pieces. Fill the measuring cup and reserve the rest for later. Set aside.

Wash the apricot and cut in half. Remove the pit and cut into bite-sized pieces. Set aside.

Peel the ginger knob and set aside.

Now, combine papaya, mango, apricot, and ginger in a juicer and process until juiced. Transfer to a serving glass and stir in the coconut water.

Add some crushed ice and enjoy!

Nutritional information per serving: Kcal: 160, Protein: 1.2g, Carbs: 45.3g, Fats: 1.2g

35.   Pineapple Orange Juice

Ingredients:

1 cup of pineapple chunks

1 small orange, peeled

1 cup of blackberries

1 small peach, pitted

¼ tsp of vanilla extract

Preparation:

Cut the top of a pineapple and peel it using a sharp paring knife. Cut into small chunks and fill the measuring cup. Reserve the rest of the pineapple in a refrigerator.

Peel the orange and divide into wedges. Set aside.

Place the blackberries in a colander and rinse thoroughly under cold running water. Set aside.

Wash the peach and cut in half. Remove the pit and cut into small pieces. Set aside.

Now, combine pineapple, orange blackberries, and peach in a juicer and process until juiced.

Transfer to a serving glasses and stir in the vanilla extract. Add few ice cubes and serve immediately.

Nutritional information per serving: Kcal: 184, Protein: 5g, Carbs: 59.2g, Fats: 1.3g

36.   Carrot Zucchini Juice

Ingredients:

1 large carrot, sliced

1 small zucchini, chopped

1 small green apple, cored

1 whole lemon, peeled

¼ tsp of ginger, ground

Preparation:

Wash and peel the carrot. Cut into thin slices and set aside.

Peel the zucchini and cut into thin slices. set aside.

Wash the apple and cut in half. Remove the core and cut into bite-sized pieces. Set aside.

Peel the lemon and cut lengthwise in half. Set aside.

Now, combine carrot, zucchini, apple, and lemon in a juicer. Process until well juiced. Transfer to a serving glass and stir in the ginger.

Add some ice and serve.

Nutritional information per serving: Kcal: 116, Protein: 3.4g, Carbs: 35.6g, Fats: 0.9g

37.   Mango Basil Juice

Ingredients:

1 whole mango, chunked

1 cup of basil, torn

4 medium-sized strawberries, chopped

1 whole kiwi, peeled

Preparation:

Peel the mango and cut into small chunks. Set aside.

Rinse the basil thoroughly under cold running water and slightly drain. Torn with hands and set aside.

Wash the strawberries and remove the stems. Cut into bite-sized pieces and set aside.

Peel the kiwi and cut lengthwise in half. Set aside.

Now, combine mango, basil, strawberries, and kiwi in a juicer and process until juiced. Transfer to a serving glass and add some ice before serving.

Enjoy!

Nutritional information per serving: Kcal: 230, Protein: 4.6g, Carbs: 64.7g, Fats: 1.9g

38.   Apple Green Tea Juice

Ingredients:

1 medium-sized Granny Smith's apple, cored

1 cup of fresh mint, torn

1 whole lemon, peeled

1 medium-sized celery stalk

1 tsp of green tea

1 tbsp of liquid honey

Preparation:

Wash the apple and cut in half. Remove the core and cut into bite-sized pieces. Set aside.

Wash the mint thoroughly under cold running water. Torn with hands and set aside.

Peel the lemon and cut lengthwise in half. Chop into quarters and set aside.

Place green tea in a small bowl. Add two tablespoons of hot water and let it soak for 5 minutes.

Wash the celery stalk and chop it into bite-sized pieces. Set aside.

Now, combine apple, mint, lemon, celery, and green tea mixture in a juicer and process until well juiced. Transfer to a serving glass and stir in the honey.

Refrigerate for 20 minutes before serving.

Nutritional information per serving: Kcal: 163, Protein: 2.6g, Carbs: 43.1g, Fats: 0.8g

39. Cranberry Orange Juice

Ingredients:

1 cup of cranberries

1 large orange, peeled

1 whole kiwi, peeled

2 whole plums, pitted

¼ tsp of cinnamon, ground

Preparation:

Place the cranberries in a colander. Wash thoroughly under cold water and slightly drain. Set aside.

Peel the orange and divide into wedges. Cut each wedge in half and set aside.

Peel the kiwi and cut lengthwise in half. Set aside.

Wash the plums and cut each in half. Remove the pits and cut into bite-sized pieces. Set aside.

Now, combine cranberries, orange, kiwi, and plums in a juicer and process until juiced. Transfer to a serving glass and stir in the cinnamon.

Add some ice and serve immediately.

Nutritional information per serving: Kcal: 182, Protein: 3.8g, Carbs: 59.1g, Fats: 1.1g

40.   Pepper Kale Juice

Ingredients:

1 medium-sized red bell pepper, chopped

1 cup of fresh kale, torn

1 cup of fresh spinach, torn

1 large radish, sliced

1 cup of cucumber, sliced

1 oz. of water

Preparation:

Wash the bell pepper and cut lengthwise in half. Remove the seeds and cut into small pieces. Set aside.

Combine kale and spinach in a colander. Wash thoroughly under cold running water and slightly drain. Torn with hands and set aside.

Wash the radish and trim off the green parts. Cut into thin slices and set aside.

Wash the cucumber and cut into thin slices. Fill the measuring cup and reserve the rest for later.

Now, combine bell pepper, kale, spinach, radish, and cucumber in a juicer and process until juiced.

Transfer to a serving glass and stir in the water. Refrigerate for 10 minutes before serving.

Enjoy!

Nutritional information per serving: Kcal: 86, Protein: 10.5g, Carbs: 22.8g, Fats: 1.9g

41.   Peach Pineapple Juice

Ingredients:

1 medium-sized peach, chopped

1 cup of pineapple, chunked

1 small zucchini, cut into bite-sized pieces

¼ tsp of ginger, ground

2 tbsp. of coconut water

Preparation:

Wash the peach and cut in half. Remove the pit and cut into bite-sized pieces. Set aside.

Using a sharp paring knife, cut the top of the pineapple. Gently remove all hard skin and slice it into thin slices. Fill the measuring cup and reserve the rest for later.

Wash the zucchini and cut into bite-sized pieces. Set aside.

Now, combine peach, pineapple, and zucchini in a juicer and process until well juiced. Transfer to a serving glass and stir in the ginger and coconut water.

Refrigerate for 10 minutes before serving.

Enjoy!

Nutritional information per serving: Kcal: 141, Protein: 3.7g, Carbs: 41.6g, Fats: 0.9g

42. Mango Strawberry Juice

Ingredients:

1 cup of mango, chunked

½ cup of strawberries, cut into bite-sized pieces

1 small apple, cored

2 whole cherries, pitted

1 tsp of dried mint, ground

Preparation:

Peel the mango and cut into bite-sized pieces. Set aside.

Wash the strawberries and remove the core. Cut into bite-sized pieces and set aside.

Wash the apple and cut in half. Remove the core and cut into small pieces. Set aside.

Wash the cherries and cut each in half. Remove the pits and set aside.

Place the mint in a small bowl and add two tablespoons of hot water. Let it soak for 5 minutes.

Now, combine mango, strawberries, apple, cherries and mint mixture in a juicer and process until juiced. Transfer to a serving glass and refrigerate for 15 minutes before serving.

Enjoy!

Nutritional information per serving: Kcal: 185, Protein: 2.8g, Carbs: 53.8g, Fats: 1.1g

43. Pomegranate Beet Juice

Ingredients:

2 cups of pomegranate seeds

1 cup of beets, sliced

1 cup of watercress, chopped

1 cup of fresh basil, chopped

¼ tsp of ginger, ground

Preparation:

For two cups of pomegranate seeds, you'll need about two medium-sized pomegranate fruits. First, cut the top of each pomegranate fruit using a sharp paring knife. Slice down to each of the white membranes inside of the fruit. Pop the seeds into a measuring cups and set aside.

Wash the beets and trim off green ends. Chop into bite-sized pieces and fill the measuring cup. Reserve the rest for later.

Combine watercress and basil in a colander. Rinse thoroughly under cold running water. Drain and roughly chop it. Set aside.

Now, combine pomegranate seeds, beets, watercress, and basil in a juicer and process until well juiced. Transfer to a serving glass and stir in the ginger.

Refrigerate for 10 minutes before serving.

Enjoy!

Nutritional information per serving: Kcal: 166, Protein: 6.6g, Carbs: 46.6g, Fats: 2.5g

44.   Melon Parsnip Juice

Ingredients:

1 large wedge of honeydew melon

1 cup of parsnips, sliced

1 medium-sized carrot, sliced

1 cup of cucumber, sliced

¼ tsp of ginger, ground

Preparation:

Cut one large honeydew melon wedge and peel it. Remove the seeds and cut into bite-sized pieces. Wrap the rest of the melon in a plastic foil and refrigerate.

Wash and slightly peel the parsnips. Cut into thin slices and fill the measuring cup. Reserve the rest for later. Set aside.

Wash and peel the carrot. Cut into thin slices and set aside.

Wash the cucumber and cut into slices. Fill the measuring cup and reserve the rest for later.

Now, combine melon, parsnips, carrot, and cucumber in a juicer and process until juiced. Transfer to a serving glass and stir in the ginger. Refrigerate for 10 minutes before serving.

Enjoy!

Nutritional information per serving: Kcal: 152, Protein: 3.4g, Carbs: 46.2g, Fats: 0.9g

ADDITIONAL TITLES FROM THIS AUTHOR

70 Effective Meal Recipes to Prevent and Solve Being Overweight: Burn Fat Fast by Using Proper Dieting and Smart Nutrition

By

Joe Correa CSN

48 Acne Solving Meal Recipes: The Fast and Natural Path to Fixing Your Acne Problems in Less Than 10 Days!

By

Joe Correa CSN

41 Alzheimer's Preventing Meal Recipes: Reduce or Eliminate Your Alzheimer's Condition in 30 Days or Less!

By

Joe Correa CSN

70 Effective Breast Cancer Meal Recipes: Prevent and Fight Breast Cancer with Smart Nutrition and Powerful Foods

By

Joe Correa CSN

www.ingramcontent.com/pod-product-compliance
Lightning Source LLC
Chambersburg PA
CBHW030246030426
42336CB00009B/281